FAT LOSS 2-4-6

Lose up to 2 Dress Sizes

Using 4 Simple Keys

in Just 6 Weeks

Naima S

ISBN-13: 978-1508697947

ISBN-10: 1508697949

http://naima.co

To the audaciously awesome biker chicks of Ankara. You rock.

Contents

About This Book

The idea for this book came to me some years ago.

It was early September, and still insanely hot and humid in the Emirates.

Co-workers were trickling in from their summer vacations that week. Some tanned and well rested, others a little exhausted from doing the usual rounds with family and relatives.

As expatriates working in Dubai, a portion of summer holidays were always earmarked to go back to our home country, and spend some time with the extended family, especially so when showing off how much the little ones had grown since the last visit home.

But the one thing all returning vacationers had in common was this: we all brought back some extra weight.

Holding my cup of green tea, I was commiserating with our office manager, Rachel, over the 8-10 pounds that once again appeared over the summer holidays, courtesy of our respective mother-in-laws, both of whom happen to be fantastic cooks.

We had both been back just over six weeks, and she was asking me how I managed to dump the extra weight so quickly.

"Well, it wasn't really that quick," I told her. "I started the day I got back, and it's been about 6 weeks."

"But what did you do?"

I explained my little secret to her. Actually, it's not really a secret.

It is mostly common sense, coupled with attention to timing and sprinkled with lots of cheat options, so that it is sustainable.

Fast forward a couple of months, and Rachel was back into her favourite black trousers, the ones she couldn't begin to zip up, much less wear comfortably.

This book lays out the keys of what worked for me and worked for Rachel in dumping those extra pounds so I could get back into my pre-holiday clothes — without struggling.

Disclaimer: I'm not a doctor, a dietician, a nutritionist or any kind of specialist, and make no claims whatsoever to that effect. The contents of this book are simply my experiences, and not to be deemed as advice. Continue reading at your own risk!

Be sensible: consult with your health practitioner before embarking on any new program, ok?

Right, with that out of the way, let's also take a moment to talk about who **this book is NOT for**:

- You have a medical condition that necessitates a special diet.

- You have more than 50 pounds to lose. This book might still help you, but there are probably better options for you.

- You are not interested in sticking with anything for longer than three days.

- You are looking for an overnight miracle.

- You believe that pills, exercise or both can compensate for a bad diet.

Still here? Excellent.

This book is for you if:

- You need to deal with those last 10 pounds that

are stubbornly hanging on.

- You are happy to try just about anything — within reason — for a few weeks, especially if you see results.

- You understand the power of slow and steady winning the race, and believe in the power of the compound effect.

- You have a killer outfit you've been dying to get back into.

- You can't stand the idea of measuring, counting and generally depriving yourself.

So, sit back, relax, and read on for the fat loss 2-4-6 formula that helped me dump two dress sizes in six weeks.

Introduction

"Successful weight loss requires programming, not will power"

- Phil McGraw

Like me, you have probably devoured (excuse the term!) dozens of how-to guides on shedding some weight.

Like me, you've probably not been entirely successful, consistent or happy with any of them.

I would also guess that, like me, fitting in calorie counting, shopping for exotic spices, and goodness, the latest in Zumba or kettle workouts don't quite overwhelm you with enthusiasm.

Well, you're in luck.

I'm about to share an approach with you which has

helped me get down from a size 14 to a size 8 in just a few weeks. Actually, six weeks to be exact.

True, I wasn't massively overweight to begin with, but like anyone in my situation will tell you, the last 10 pounds are an absolute nightmare to get rid of.

The cool thing is that they came off without devoting inordinate amounts of time to "45-60 minutes of cardio, 5 to 6 times a week". Yikes. Who actually even has that much time to just spend on themselves?

I will tell you, though, that you will have to make *some* changes. However, they are not massive, going-to-India-to-find-myself kind of changes.

Some will be tough initially, for about 3-4 days. Then they will become easy. Really.

Other changes will be easy and so blindingly obvious, that after you start to make them, you will wonder why you you didn't think of them yourself.

But the best part of it all is that the changes are simple.

Because they are simple, you might think that they don't do the job and won't work. Trust me, complexity doesn't always equal effectiveness.

But because they are so simple, and require practically

no preparation, you will be able to easily incorporate them into your day-to-day life.

So, without further ado, let us delve in.

The Four Keys

"Stressed spelled backwards is desserts. Coincidence? I think not!"

— Unknown

Before getting to the four keys, let me start by telling you that I read a lot.

Books. Blogs. Back of packages. Podcasts - technically, that's not reading, but you get the picture. I totally overdose on research.

I also like to experiment, especially when it comes to looking and feeling great.

You see, I'm inherently lazy, impatient and vain. This is a deadly combination, but the right one that motivated me to research, experiment, and finally extract the shortest, least painful route to fat loss that works, works fast, and doesn't require that I do a ton of preparation work.

True, there are way too many variables to fat loss for non-Tim-Ferriss individuals to figure out. After all, not all of us are predisposed to run labs on ourselves every other day while experimenting.

But we all know the basics. More or less.

In digging through and trying to figure out what works best for individuals like me (little time, even less will power, wants results NOW), I discovered that four factors kept coming up time and again.

I found that handled the right way, these four keys in the right combination open the elusive fat loss door.

No need to hold your breath - it's nothing earth shatteringly new, nor is it rocket science.

The four keys are: Hydration, Nutrition, Metabolism, and Rest.

But - the trick is in approaching them just the right way.

In other words, in a way that doesn't require large amounts of willpower, discipline, tons of measuring and all of the other annoying activities usually associated with a weight loss program.

So let's go through each of these keys in turn, understand their impact on fat loss, and how to tweak them to do our bidding.

Key #1 - Hydration

"Pure water is the world's first and foremost medicine."

— Slovakian Proverb

Hydration is a word used to describe the body's ability to manage water. Of course, we all know how important water is. It's a no brainer that hydration is essential for good health.

What is good hydration?

Let me put it this way: if you get thirsty, it's your body's way of telling you it is already reached some level of dehydration.

For our purposes, we want to keep well hydrated for one simple reason: when the body senses impending dehydration, it starts shutting off what it considers superfluous functions, and it focuses on keeping us alive.

As an aside, stress has a similar effect, in that any function that doesn't help fight or flight, is basically put aside.

Guess what fits into the category of non-critical functions? Waste elimination.

So no matter what kind of diet you go on, or how hard you work out, unless you are well hydrated, you will not eliminate fat.

It also means that unless you are taking in enough water, your energy levels will be low as the body is focusing on preserving what little hydration is left.

The impact of low energy is that you will reach for the nearest boost - coffee, a chocolate bar and so on, because your will power will also be low.

This entire counter-productive domino effect can be avoided by just making water an intrinsic part of your life.

It is also a well known fact that we often mistake thirst signals for hunger. We eat when we really need to drink water.

If you're still not convinced, let me share this little tidbit with you: a clinical research centre in Germany found that after just 17 ounces of water, metabolism goes up by 30 percent!

This means you could drink a little over two cups of water and have your metabolism respond almost immediately.

Your body is made of 60-70% water. Follow these guidelines to keep it that way:

- Start your day with 1-2 glasses of water as soon as you wake up. No, not an hour later. As soon as you wake up.

- Try to drink cold water whenever possible. It will jolt your metabolism as it scrambles to re-heat you to normal temperature.

- Drink a glass of water 30 minutes before every meal. It will help you feel full faster when you do eat.

- Replace sodas, fruit juices and other empty, sweet drinks with water. If you can't stand the sheer boredom and blandness of water, add a tiny amount of your favourite sports drink, just enough to flavour it.

- Fizzy water with a bit of lemon can feel very

glamorous to sip throughout the day.

- Get a cool glass or an even cooler bottle to keep in your bag, on your desk or in your sports bag.

- Learn to make and enjoy refreshing green smoothies with just vegetables and cold water. They are fantastic for cleansing you and eliminating the junk that clogs up your fat burning equipment, such as your liver.

As you start to ramp up your water intake towards the 2-3 litres per day, you will be having a fun time with your bladder, but only while your body adjusts to your new water levels.

Don't let the prospect of frequent urination get in the way of your hydration.

However, be smart and know when to slow down your water intake if you know you won't have access to washrooms easily.

Similarly, try to get most of your water in before 7 pm so that you can flush out your bladder before bed and get an uninterrupted night's sleep.

Important: don't overdo the water intake. If that's all you are drinking, as in you are not eating or drinking anything else, make sure you include a pinch of salt every now and again. The last you want to do is to upset the electrolyte balance in your body, which could be lead to potentially dangerous conditions such as water intoxication (yes, it's a thing):

"The issue boils down to sodium levels. One of sodium's jobs is to balance the fluids in and around your cells. Drinking too much water causes an imbalance, and the liquid moves from your blood to inside your cells, making them swell. Swelling inside the brain is serious and requires immediate treatment." WebMD.

Keep it under a litre per hour, and you should be fine.

Hydration Checklist

Use the list below to orient yourself in the morning, and as a checklist in the evening to see if you were able to use the hydration key to your advantage:

- I drank water as soon as I got out bed

- I drank water before most of my meals

- I did not feel thirsty

- I drank clear or green liquids 80% of the time

- I did not consume any sweet drinks

- I consumed approximately 2 litres of clean liquids

Key #2 - Nutrition

"The food you eat can be either the safest and most powerful form of medicine or the slowest form of poison."

— Ann Wigmore

We all know what nutrition is, right? It's the fuel that we put into our body to give it the energy it needs to function so we can walk, play, work, live ...

Nutrition is supposed to give us nutrients. Sadly, most nutrition plans - our meals - are neither planned, nor nutritious. They are high in quantity, but low in quality for the most part.

Let's start with sugar and its substitutes. You know and I know that taste, and particularly a sweet tooth, is a learned thing.

Nobody was born craving a Diet Coke or a Twinkie. We learned to like it. We learned to prefer bread and pasta over broccoli and spinach.

While I wouldn't go so far as to suggest that you unlearn how to like pizza and ice cream, I will propose to you the notion that you can totally control your taste buds.

You see, it's all about having the right frame of reference.

For example, if you eat a piece of cabbage, then follow that up with a banana, you will notice how sweet the banana is.

On the other hand, if you eat ice cream, then eat the same banana, suddenly the banana won't seem as sweet.

Our base reference for what is "sweet" has increased so much over the years, that we could be practically eating a teaspoon of sugar, and still not find it sweet enough!

The nutrition key for our quest in weight loss is going to be to kill our addiction to sugar.

Wait - before you throw away the book in disgust - we are going to give up sugar for six days a week.

Then, on our seventh day, or cheat day as many call it,

we're going to overload on anything that we didn't have during the week.

During the week, no sugar, no sugar substitutes, no fruit (except tomatoes and avocados).

Zero Sugar

Why are we stopping all sugar?

Sugar triggers an insulin response, a hormone that helps regulate blood sugar.

Think of insulin as this little old lady that goes around collecting any fat it can get its hands on, and takes it straight to storage, tucking it away for a rainy day.

How does fat get into our body in the first place, assuming we are not consuming pints of lard? Gosh, isn't that visual frighteningly brutal!

Eeew.

Anyway, back to insulin. Any fuel that is not used up, meaning, it is not burned and used for your normal daily functions, gets converted to fat.

I would wager that we consume way more fuel than we need, and the fastest one that gets converted to fat is sugar.

So, we lose the sugar first.

My experience has been that I crave sugar in my tea on Monday morning. By Tuesday lunchtime I don't have cravings anymore.

I've decided that I can handle that 24-30 hour period just fine, because I love the results.

Giving up sugar and fruits during the week has given me this sense of alertness and energy throughout the day that I definitely don't have when I'm indulging my taste buds with sweet stuff - sugar, sugar substitutes and fruit.

White Carbs

The other sugar-like thing we must give up six days a week is white carbohydrates, as well as anything that could be white.

This includes pasta, rice, bread and their various derivatives. And yes, this includes whole wheat pasta and brown rice. Stay away from all these carbs for the week.

Remember, you get to have them on your cheat day!

Why avoid these carbs?

The reason is that, next to sugar and fructose (from fruits), carbohydrates get quickly converted to glucose, and, if found in excess of what is required for the body, get converted to fat and stored by our good friend insulin.

For me, the craving for pasta (I adore the stuff) is also gone by Tuesday lunchtime, provided I eat *enough*.

Eating Enough

The big problem with no carb or low carb diets, or any diet for that matter, is that you don't eat enough.

Seriously.

Of course, if you eat half what you normally do by virtue of eliminating carbs, the calories will drop, you will experience a short term weight drop.

Then, you will plateau and start to put weight on again while still on the same diet.

Sound familiar?

The reason is because by restricting the amount calories

you consume, you send a signal to your metabolism that there's less coming in. Your metabolism reacts by slowing down, especially for women.

You look at the scale, and eat even less the next day. Your metabolism slows down even more to match the lower calorie level you are subjecting your body to.

It's a vicious circle, which usually ends in a major binge, throwing away the work done thus far, and deciding no diet will ever work.

You can neatly side step this cycle, and stick it out, and stop your metabolism from slowing down.

You just need to eat enough.

The trick is to load up, but on a different type of carbohydrates: slow carbs. These carbs that have two qualities:

- They are very high in fibre

- They take longer to break down

These wonderful carbohydrates do exist and they are called legumes or pulses. They include all kinds of beans, lentils, chick peas and so on.

Add massive amounts of pulses to your meals and you will find that not only do you feel fuller for longer, but you will have boundless energy, in a way you could never have on low carb diets.

The added fibre does not "count" towards calories as it goes right through your system, and it also keeps you, to put it delicately, regularly cleansed.

To stay full longer, use good fats liberally, such as olive oil, coconut oil, and our recently "forgiven" butter. Yes, apparently butter is now good for us. Stick to the no-additive, organic, grass-fed kind for feeling extra virtuous.

And stay away from margarine. That stuff will kill you.

Seriously. Leave out a tub of margarine, and not even flies will touch it. Food for thought, right?

For accelerating fat loss, also avoid dairy, as the lactose in milk and its derivatives seems to trigger an insulin response as well.

Cheat Day

Having a cheat day built into your program does two things:

- Gives you that light at the end of tunnel that sustains you throughout the week

- The high calorie spike stops your metabolism from "noticing" your drop in calories and adjusting down

Talk about killing two stones with one day! (sounds much nicer that killing the poor bird ...)

There are no rules for cheat day. Eat whatever you like. In whatever quantities you like. Ice cream. Pasta. Pastries. Whatever you want.

Yes, the scale will have disturbing numbers the morning after cheat day, but will quickly recover within 24-48 hours.

Which reminds me ...

Keep Track

Weigh yourself every single morning.

Of course, it would be best if had a gadget that could simply start beeping when you've reached your limit of consumption, just like at a gas distributor, the pump stops automatically.

Until someone invents one (Apple, hurry up!), you will have to do this getting in touch with your body yourself.

Start by getting on that scale every morning. Make the scale your friend, one you hang out with every day.

This kind of daily feedback loop will help you in two ways:

- Know where you stand

- Get you a little bit closer to realizing the effect of the day before's nutrition.

- Understand how you may or may not retain water

- Get you over your fear of weighing yourself

- Stop your denial

I read somewhere that this guy lost a ton of weight (not literally a ton) by just weighing himself every day.

In fact, a study conducted by the Annals of Behavioral Medicine found that "... *those who weighed themselves on a daily basis lost an average of 12 pounds, compared to people who weighed themselves weekly and lost an average of six pounds. Those who said they never weighed themselves gained an average of four pounds.*"

Crazy.

But it makes sense.

Think of those road signs that displays your speed as you approach them. You automatically slow down, right?

It's the same when you weigh yourself every day. Your subconscious gets briefed, and you will automagically eat less.

Really. Try it. For best results, use a scale that has at least one decimal point, so you can track the effect of saying no to that last snack before bed.

Nutrition Checklist

Use the guidelines below to orient yourself to what you should eat, and gradually incorporate these guidelines into your daily checklist.

- I have eliminated 90% of sugar from my meals and snacks

- I have eaten enough today and I'm not hungry

- I have eliminated rice, pasta and bread from my meals and snacks

- I have planned a great cheat day this weekend

- I have eliminated 90% of dairy from my nutrition

- I have eliminated 90% of fruit from weekday nutrition

- I have added pulses and lots of vegetables to my meals

- I weighed myself this morning

Key #3 - Metabolism

"If it weren't for the fact that the TV set and the refrigerator are so far apart, some of us wouldn't get any exercise at all."

— Joey Adams

Metabolism is complex, and well beyond the scope of this book to explain in detail.

For our purposes, it suffices to define it as the amount of energy the body burns to maintain itself.

The body is constantly burning calories - while you walk, sleep, eat, play ... it is constantly burning calories to keep you functioning.

One thing that affects your metabolism is the amount of muscle you carry. The more muscle, the more energy you burn — even while you sleep.

For example, for two people with exactly the same height and weight, the one with more muscle has a higher metabolism.

This is why, when looking to exercise, choose resistance, body weight exercises or weight training over cardio whenever possible so you can build muscle.

Quickly working through one resistance exercise after another will also give you the aerobic benefits of cardio, as you are keeping your heart rate consistently raised throughout.

On top of that of course, you get the nice side effects of building tight little muscles that burn calories in your sleep. So whenever given a choice, go for resistance.

The other thing that raises metabolism, albeit for a short period, is the actual exercise itself.

Everyone knows that you burn more calories while you exercise.

What might not be so common knowledge is that your metabolism stays raised for up to several hours afterwards, depending on the intensity of your workout.

For example, instead of 30 minutes in one block of exercise, go for 3 short sessions of 10 minutes each.

Not only will your metabolism be raised during the combined 30 minutes, but it will also remain raised for a while after each short burst, resulting in an overall longer period, during which your metabolism is working harder.

Sneaky Exercise

Speaking about exercise, I'm sure that the biggest barrier, apart from time, is *preparing* to exercise: change into the right gear, put on special shoes (heels don't work well for sprinting, but I suspect you knew that), optionally get in the car and get to a place (gym, park) to exercise.

That's just too hard, I hear you say.

Let me remind you that the objective is not to "go to the gym". The objective is to raise your metabolism.

Let me point out a few simple, super easy ways to do that:

- Jumping jacks: the old favourite. Just make sure you get your heels down when you land or you might injure yourself.

- Running in place: take off the Manolos for 5 minutes and use your (gasp!) bare feet to run in place.

- Knee raises: you don't even need to change shoes for this. Raise one knee as high as you can, then repeat on the other side. Quickly.

- Seated jog: great for cubicle warriors. Mimic jogging while seated. It's harder than you think!

- Pump and punch: use your arms and alternate pumping your fists up and punching in front of you. Great de-stresser when paired with a visual of your favourite personal villain on the punch part.

- Run up and down a set of stairs a few times. Run up and walk down - great high intensity interval training.

- Squats: this has got to be about the best all around exercise there is for the lower body. Spend a few minutes on YouTube to get a visual of how to do it right, and you will have a weapon for life.

- Push-ups: another five star exercise and incredibly powerful for the upper body and the core. Do them at any level and watch your body transform.

- Burpees: my personal favourite and the exercise I've been having a love/hate relationship with

for like, ever. It works just about every major
muscle in the body.

If you're not familiar with burpees, let me tell you a
couple of things about them, before I describe how to
do them.

1. Burpees make everything burn: upper body,
    lower body, core, lungs, and yes, calories.

2. Burpees can be done with no equipment and
    very little space.

3. Burpees are a combination of a squat, push-up
    and jump.

Here is an image of the sequence, or you can google
"burpee video" for a tutorial.

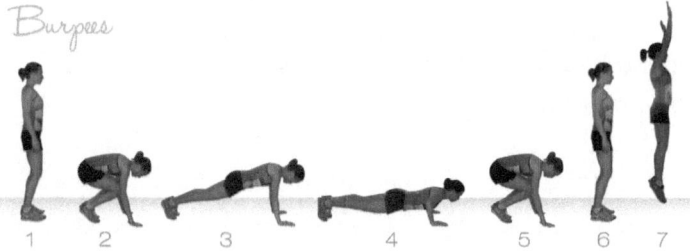

Apart from the burpees, use your imagination to come
up with fun ways to get your heart pumping a few
times throughout the day.

Before you pull out the good old "But I work in an office!" routine, let me remind you of the privacy of washroom cubicles.

You will be visiting them often anyway, what with your newly discovered commitment to hydration, right?

What is important is that you spike your metabolism at least 5 times during the day. The duration of the spike must be at least one minute.

Come on, you can do anything for just one minute!

I would personally recommend you choose strength exercises from the list mentioned above - such as squats and pushups. They are easily the most effective exercises as they recruit large and important muscle groups.

Spend half a minute doing squats, and the other half doing pushups.

Repeat for at least 5 times throughout the day, but go for 10-12 times a day if you want to see results fast.

In this way, you are keeping your metabolism elevated almost all the time. Before it gets a chance to slow back down to your resting rate, boom, here come another set of squats.

The other bonus is that you will just feel so energized throughout the whole day. Whenever you feel a tiny slump coming on, just hit the floor/wall and do 10, and you will be bursting at the seams with a sense of well being and energy.

One final tip on metabolism. This one was popularized by Tim Ferris of *The Four Hour Body* fame.

He discovered that if you do large muscle movement exercises for about 90 seconds just before a meal, and also around 90 minutes after a meal, whatever you consume tends to go to replenish energy in the muscles, rather than being sent off to be processed, likely into fat storage.

Tim also is a fan of squats and wall push-ups just before your main course is served. Another reason to disappear into a washroom cubicle at strategic moments in your day.

Don't forget to wash your hands.

Metabolism Checklist

You will be keeping your metabolism raised as much as you can during your day to keep it burning high all day. Here is the daily checklist:

- I have chosen two resistance exercises

- I managed 5-10 short bursts of exercise spread throughout the day

- I did squats and wall pushups in most of my short bursts of exercise

- I did 70-100 jumping jacks first thing this morning

- I took the stairs most of the time

Key #4 - Rest

"Sleep is that golden chain that ties health and our bodies together."

— Thomas Dekker

I keep telling my kids that they don't know it yet, because they're too young, but sleep is the most underrated activity.

There's nothing quite as satisfying, energizing and restorative as a great night of sleep, spent in deep, deep slumber.

Sleep is important, really important. They say babies do most of their growing while they sleep. We also know that most healing, body repair and rejuvenation happens during sleep.

Specifically, the liver, the organ responsible for

metabolizing fat, works primarily at night, breaking down nutrients and harmful substances alike, and processing them into their right channels.

This detoxification doesn't begin until we are at rest. It also doesn't begin if there are other active, critical processes going on, such as digesting a heavy evening meal.

For this reason, you should keep in mind that proteins take longer to digest, so allow a good 3 hours between your last meal and when you retire for the night.

When you don't get enough good quality sleep, your liver's capability to breakdown fat and toxins is heavily compromised, resulting in unwanted side effects, such as fat accumulation and severely diminished ability to efficiently process food into clean fuel.

Bottom line is, if you are interested in weight loss and overall health, make sleep a priority. Once on the slippery road to insomnia and a fatty liver, it is difficult to make a clean come back.

Rest Checklist

I won't bore you with the whole no electronics in the bedroom routine. You know the drill, but here are just a few checklist items on rest:

- I allowed 2-3 hours after dinner before bed

- I slept 7-8 hours

- I had a light meal for dinner

Incorporating The Keys

"You will never change your life until you change something you do daily. The secret of your success is found in your daily routine."

— Darren Hardy, The Compound Effect

You now have the four keys to simplified fat loss, understand how they work together, and have a daily checklist for each key to keep you on track.

Start a journal, and note your progress.

Capture what goes well, what you are struggling with.

I won't recommend that you take pictures of your meals before you have them (bit creepy, no?), but do keep track of any slips into sugar, dairy or white carbs.

It will help you understand what your scale and the fit

of your jeans are telling you.

You can use the day-by-day guideline below to kickstart your program and your journal.

Day One

Pick one or two items from each checklist, and commit to it each day. Water and squats every time you use the washroom are good and easy starting points. Feel good about the success. Especially the squats.

Day Two

Pick out another set of items from the checklists to try. Ignore the little headache. It's your toxins begging you for sugar. Notice the tingling in your muscles from yesterday's bursts of exercises. Feel great.

Day Three

On day three, when your resolve is about waver, think about what you will have for breakfast on your cheat day. Drink some cold water and persevere. You have already invested 2.5 days. Might as well stick with it. Go on, do another squat or two while you're waiting for the shower to heat up.

Day Four

You are now past hump day. Add a few more items

from the checklist. Try a new lentil recipe to make up
for the tiny slip at lunch time (toasted bread doesn't
count as real bread, right? Wrong.) Repent for 90
seconds and move on. Congratulate yourself for hitting
8 bursts of exercise today.

Day Five

Wake up refreshed and incredulous at how well you
slept. Have spinach soup with a tablespoon of flaxseed
for breakfast without even glancing at the cereal box.
(Note: soup for breakfast is amazing).

Grin to yourself and wonder if it really is this easy. Yes,
it is.

Day Six

Last day of the week. Marvel at how great green tea
tastes without sugar. Have a throw-everything-in salad
with a simple vinaigrette, and go to sleep with a massive
smile on your face, dreaming of a rich, creamy lasagna.

Day Seven

Wake up on Cheat Day and head for the scale. Yell
"YES!" and pump your fist up in the air. Drink some
cold water, and start your systematic devouring of all
the chocolate you saved up all week.

Congratulations. You did it. You got results by tweaking a tiny bit at a time. Your consistency has paid off.

Wrap Up

"The big secret in life is that there is no big secret. Whatever your goal, you can get there if you are willing to work."

-Oprah Winfrey

Weight loss is really not that complicated.

We make it complicated when we look for ways to absolve ourselves of responsibility for getting fat.

You now know the four keys to uncomplicated, simple and sustainable fat loss. To summarize:

- Drink lots of water, preferably cold, and always first thing upon waking

- Stay away from bread, pasta, rice, dairy, sugar and fruit for six days a week

- Eat plenty of pulses instead, as well as protein and vegetables until you are full

- Spike your metabolism by doing 5-10 spurts of 1-2 minutes of exercise throughout the day, preferably squats and pushups

- Get some reasonable sleep

- Weigh and measure yourself on the morning of cheat day, track and celebrate your results

Rejoice in the knowledge that you have the power to lose weight at will.

You made the choice when you got this book, and you will make the right choice again right now when you get started.

Once you decide, truly decide, to take charge of your body, and follow these key principles, fat loss is simple, sustainable and completely within your control.

Enjoy your newly tweaked body!

Want Some More?

Thank you for reading this guide. I hope you enjoyed it and came away with some insights into how you can tackle getting down a size or two in a simple, no-fuss and effective manner.

I like to write pragmatic guides on mindset, productivity and feeling great — inside and out.

If you would like to know when my next book is out, and also be notified of promotions and the free downloads I often run, you might want to join my mailing list.

Just go over to naima.co/signup to sign up.

Just One More Thing

I always appreciate feedback.

I thank you in advance for taking the time to let me know of any errors, omissions, or other things you feel detract from the book. You can find me at naima@naima.co.

In a moment, Amazon and your e-reader will prompt you for a review. I would be most grateful if you could spare a few minutes to write a review, however short. You can always add to it later.

Your review will help this book become visible to others who might benefit from it, and help me go just a tiny bit further in my quest of living the digital life.

Thank you!

My Other Books

You can find my other books at my author page on
Amazon:

http://naima.co/authorpage

I write about productivity, motivation, feeling great and
a host of other things as I learn and live them.

About The Author

My name is Naima, and I'm a grown-up third culture kid.

I was born in London to Somali parents, studied in Africa, Europe, Asia and America, which meant I had to learn a few languages … fast.

Fun fact: I was also once run over by a cow. I survived, but for a bruised ego.

I love to write and all things digital, both of which I've had a love affair with for a few decades - way before it was cool to know how to code. Yes, I'm that young.

I currently live in Turkey with my Italian husband and our two teenage kids — both of whom were born in the United Arab Emirates — extending the third culture life for another generation.

You can contact me directly on naima@naima.co or find me in any of the following places:

Blog: http://naima.co/blog

Twitter: http://twitter.com/_naima

Linkedin: http://linkedin.com/in/naimadotco